Knees *for*
LIFE

Leading
self-treatment
method to
end knee pain

BILL PARRAVANO

"I've had the pleasure of speaking with Bill about my own knee injury, and his knowledge in the area is incredible. My knees have been incredibly healthy all my life, despite being active in sports and bodybuilding; yet at almost 50, I know I need to be more proactive at keeping them that way. That's why I recommend Bill's book. If you want healthy knees, this is your go-to guide."

Jon Dana Benson
4-time Bestselling Fitness/Nutrition Author
CEO, Fitology
www.Fitology.com

"Bill Parravano's approach to reversing knee pain is strategic, smart, and remarkably effective. Rather than treating symptoms, he helps you to address the underlying causes of the knee pain you're dealing with. What you learn in this book will empower you to have healthy, functional knees for the rest of your life."

Shawn Stevenson
Fitness & Nutrition Expert
www.TheFatLossCode.com

"Bill Parravano's comprehensive knowledge and understanding of the knee and how it connects to the rest of your body is revolutionary. Worried you'll live with knee pain forever? This holistic approach to healing knee pain will make your worries obsolete."

Jena la Flamme
Pleasurable Weight Loss Expert,
www.PleasurableWeightLoss.com

"Knees for Life is a must read for anyone who has ever heard, "In a few years you'll be a perfect candidate for a knee replacement."

Dr. Paul Constante
www.dynamicmedrehab.com

"Bill Parravano is quite simply a gifted healer. He took my knee in his hands and started to move it around with the skill of a true professional. In moments, years of uncomfortable knee pain started to disappear. He explains everything in easy terms and showed me that the body has an amazing ability to heal itself."

Emmanuel Manolakakis
Owner and Chief Instructor
FightClub Martial Arts & Fitness Training Centre Inc.
www.Fight-Club.ca

"For anyone suffering from chronic knee pain, this book will be a godsend, because in it not only will Bill show you how to get out of pain now, but he'll also teach you how to preserve your knees for the long haul. As a professional peer, I had always admired Bill Parravano's work, but it wasn't until I had my own issues with pain that I learned what an incredibly gifted healer he truly is. Simply put, his techniques work like magic! I cannot recommend his work more highly."

Eve Colantoni
CHC Certified Health, Wellness and Nutrition Coach
National Integrated Health Associates (NIHA)
www.NIHAdc.com

Knees for Life
Leading Self-Treatment Method to End Knee Pain
Bill Parravano

Copyright© 2013
ISBN Print: 9780615842660
ISBN Digital: 9780615842666

The information provided in this book is designed to provide helpful information on the subjects discussed. This book is not meant to be used, nor should it be used, to diagnose or treat any medical condition. For diagnosis or treatment of any medical problem, consult your own physician. The publisher and author are not responsible for any specific health needs that may require medical supervision and are not liable for any damages or negative consequences from any treatment, action, application or preparation to any person reading or following the information in this book. References are provided for informational purposes only and do not constitute endorsement of any websites or other sources. Readers should be aware that the websites listed in this book may change.

Published by
Bill Parravano
P.O. Box 2413
Asheville, NC 28802

Printed in the United States of America

DEDICATION

This book is dedicated to my daughter. May the work I do today create a better world for you to live in.

TABLE OF CONTENTS

FOREWORD
Bo Eason

There's a saying in the NFL that goes like this: "If you can't play, you can't stay." Truer words were never spoken!

I remember lying atop a table inside the Houston Oilers training room in 1987, my knee packed in ice after my seventh knee surgery. Those words echoed through my head, "If you can't play, you can't stay."

Sounds harsh, but is it any different than your life today? I think, not.

We live in a performance-based world.

Think back over your life—every success, every failure, every promotion or demotion, every raise or cut in pay you've received is based on your performance.

If you're unable to perform, you will be left behind.

Today, I make my living speaking on stages around the world. Again, my job, like yours, is performance based.

Last year, I was in Los Angeles, training a group of professionals. I was on my feet, onstage, all day. At the end of the day, I headed backstage, where I was stopped by a man who said, "I can help you with the knee pain you're experiencing." I couldn't believe it. As a former NFL player, I pride myself on not showing any pain. But, there was no hiding pain from this man. I asked, "How'd you know?" He calmly said, "Some things are unmistakable to me. Knee pain is one of them. I can help you."

I was in a hurry and wanted nothing more than to get off my feet, but the man and I agreed to talk at a dinner function later that night.

Later, at the dinner party, I was making the rounds to each table, visiting and taking photos when I ran into the knee-pain man again. He said, "Sit down at my table for a minute." So, I sat down. Without a word, he took hold of my ankle and foot, lifted them up onto his knees. He began to apply steady, firm pressure onto my lower leg. After 30 seconds, I could feel heat in my knee and a relief that I hadn't felt for 30 years.

After a couple of minutes, the man had me stand up. The heat had spread throughout my whole leg by then. It's hard to explain the exact sensation in words, but I felt as if I was standing on top of my leg for the first time. For the first time, the structure and stability of my knee felt sound and secure. And the best part was, no pain.

I immediately turned to the man and asked, "What's your name?" He said, "Bill Parravano!"

As you might guess, Bill Parravano is one of my most favorite people in the world.

Thanks to Bill Parravano, I get to continue to perform at the highest level, and so can you.

Bill Parravano wrote this book, *Knees for Life,* so you and I will never have to hear or fear those words again, "If you can't play, you can't stay."

INTRODUCTION

My mission is to make knee-replacement surgery obsolete.

Whether most people with chronic knee pain know it or not, they are likely on a slippery slope to knee-replacement surgery, no matter what their current diagnosis. The current and conventional approach to knee pain typically leads to surgical replacement of the joint. By following the *Knees for Life* protocol, you will save yourself years of undue suffering, a possible reliance on prescription drugs, painful injections in the knee joint, and time and money spent on physical therapy.

It's important to know who you are trusting regarding knee-pain advice and how to create the prime conditions that will allow your body to heal itself. You might be asking, "Who is this guy and why should I listen to him?" You'll soon learn of my personal background, my extensive training, hands-on experience, and my own journey with knee-pain. My no-nonsense approach reaches most knee conditions. Experiencing knee pain and seeking help to relieve it can seem like a dead-end street, where you might feel like you ask the same questions and hear the same ineffective answers—all while your knee pain worsens. I will show you how to avoid things that simply don't work. Using my approach, you will be able to utilize the most effective techniques to get out of knee pain fast.

I want to thank you in advance for taking the time to read this book. I applaud your commitment; taking this leap forward can be downright terrifying if you are already in pain. By beginning this healing journey, you are going to be moving toward regaining the knees you had when you were younger, and right now is the best time to get started.

■ ■ ■

Before we begin, please go to my website,
www.KneesForLife.com,
and sign up for my newsletter.
You will receive updated news and assistance on
eliminating your chronic knee pain.

Chapter 1

I'VE WALKED (AND LIMPED) IN YOUR SHOES

Why can I help (and relate to) you on a level that most physical therapists and doctors cannot? I have personally lived through four knee dislocations and a resulting ACL reconstruction—and have also had two pieces of meniscus taken out of my knee. The prescription drugs given to me to numb the pain only made me violently ill and masked the pain. Due to my own fear of potential surgery, I was unable to relieve my knee pain for almost two years, because under no circumstances did I want to have a future knee-replacement surgery. To find an alternative to surgery, I had to find the solution to pain-free knees through my own extensive research and training.

My Training and Background

I've completed 2,000 hours (and counting) of practitioner training under the Society of Ortho Bionomy® International. Ortho Bionomy® is an osteopathic-based style of healing which places the body, first and foremost, in a state of comfort to accelerate the release of pain and tension. I have also been studying, training, and instructing a Russian style of martial arts called Systema for over 13 years. Systema focuses on breathing, building strong joints, and a healthy body. I have traveled the globe, researching real-world experiences and seeking the truth to find what will help both me and my clients. I've worked with all ages and conditions: from teenagers to adults to seniors; all had diagnoses varying in complexity, from sprained knees, arthritic knee joints, to bone-on-bone situations. The cornerstone of my approach is the simple, yet profound, wisdom that the body has the capacity and ability to heal itself. You just have to work with your body, not against it. My job is to show you how.

What Drives Me to Help You

Whether or not most knee-pain sufferers realize it, they are on a downward spiral to knee-replacement surgery (a conventional medical approach to chronic knee pain). It's insane that drugs, pain-killing injections, and "exploratory" surgeries are the only options available until you are old enough (or degenerated enough) to have knee-replacement surgery, where bones are cut and removed in the leg and replaced with plastic and metal. This isn't the only solution, and that's what motivates me to help you. I see it time and time again with clients who have been diagnosed with bone-on-bone scenarios: they can regain comfort and mobility in their body without surgery and live fulfilling lives as a result.

Knees for Life is for anyone who is looking "outside the box" for solutions to escape the cycle of drugs, shots, and surgery. It's for someone with an open mind, who is willing to put 30 minutes a day into making sure their knees feel pain free. What you will gain from the *Knees for Life* protocol is a template to eliminate your knee pain, repair and restore your knees, and keep those joints healthy for the rest of your life.

Now that you know a little more about my personal experience with knee pain and surgery, my training, background, and more about my perspective and approach, we can really get started. Remember, I bring years of hands-on experience, thorough research, and a strong desire and dedication to help each client reach his or her personal health goals. Keeping an open mind and setting aside a little time and dedication each day is all it will take.

If Only I'd had the Right Information...

The first time I wish I'd had this book was in December of 1998, after I arrived home from skiing with a dislocated knee. If I had had this information back then, there would have been a distinct possibility that I would never have undergone knee surgery.

The second time I wish I had this book was in June of 1999, right after I got back from ACL reconstructive surgery. These exercises, techniques, and methods would have reduced my recovery time from that surgery, and I would have been back to practicing Judo in a fraction of the time it took me to heal and regain the necessary mobility.

I call my approach "Mission Possible." In my lifetime, I want to make knee-replacement surgery obsolete. My goal is to completely change your perspective on how your body works and heals itself after implementing the *Knees for Life* approach. I want to eliminate the words "knee-replacement surgery" from your vocabulary!

■ ■ ■

ACTION STEP:

Follow me on Twitter -
http://www.Twitter.com/TheKneePainGuru *let's keep in*
touch, network, and share pertinent information.

Chapter 2

STEP BY STEP

Have you found yourself feeling confused and frustrated by what's coming out of your doctor's mouth? You're being told that nothing is wrong with your knee, yet you still have pain. Maybe you've been through X-rays, CT scans, or MRIs and been told, "There is nothing wrong with your knee." Perhaps, you have even been through a surgery to repair or replace what was broken or torn, and your doctor considers your knee to be mechanically sound, yet you still have knee pain.

The principles and tools in this book apply to people of all ages. No matter what your stage in life, all bodies work on the same principles: we need good food, water, oxygen, stretching, and strengthening of the body—in the proper order—to enjoy true health. These principles, in fact, are critical tools our bodies require to set up the prime conditions which allow the body (and our knees) to heal. Beginning with the correct mindset on this journey is crucial to ensure you get the end result you need: to be out of knee pain fast and make permanent changes. The order in which *Knees for Life* tools and principles are applied will be slightly different from person to person. Basic tools and concepts must be understood and followed so the body will be comfortable and free from pain. I've been where you are, there is a way through and out of pain; I will be there with you through this process and each step of your journey.

■ ■ ■

"You never change something by fighting the existing reality.
To change something, build a new model that makes the
existing model obsolete."
~ R. Buckminster Fuller

Chapter 3

THE OSTRICH SYNDROME

When I was 28, my friend and chiropractor, Dr. Paul, invited me to go snow skiing. I thought, *"Why not? I work out regularly, train, and compete in Judo. I'm pretty invincible."* But I hadn't skied in years, and despite being in really good physical shape, the first hop off the ski lift that day left me feeling very nervous.

Anyone who has stood atop an intimidating ski slope for the first time (or the first time in a long while) might relate to what I felt: butterflies in the stomach, body tense, sweating even though it's cold enough to snow, and then the physical sensation of the first push off and tentative creeping down the hill.

After I began my descent, my speed picked up faster than I was ready for. My body tensed up more; I held my breath. I remember thinking, *"Just go diagonally down the hill until you get used to it."* So I steered more perpendicularly left in the hope of slowing down. That's when things quickly went wrong. On the upside of the slope was powder, and on the downside of the slope was ice. My legs started doing the splits as I was trying to "snow plow" to slow myself down (if you aren't familiar with the snow plow, it's a technique used to teach beginning skiers how to slow their speed or stop.) Already going too fast, I lost my balance and fell face first into the icy snow, my legs awkwardly stretched behind me, while locked into the stiff ski boots, accompanied by an alarming amount of pain emanating from my left leg.

I remember the fall, and lying there on the ski slope just focusing on my breath to keep myself from vomiting or passing out. My ears began to ring, and my body began to shiver from the extreme cold as I was beginning to blackout. I remember feeling embarrassed as I watched little kids ski around me effortlessly, as I was taken down the mountain in the first-aid sled. Fortunately, my ski buddy, Dr. Paul, is a chiropractor and looked at my leg in the ski lodge and did a quick adjustment onsite.

That snowy day was the first of four times that I dislocated my left knee. The second episode was in Judo, and the third time was in volleyball. The fourth time, I was playing shortstop in a softball league—I heard the crack of the bat and shuffled quickly to the left toward the ball—I was on it! The ground ball was coming directly toward me. I scooped it up, pivoted quickly to throw left to first base. *POP!* In a flash, I was on the ground screaming a deep, blood-curdling scream that seared through my core. I didn't know what had just happened. It didn't make sense—how could I be in so much pain? How could my leg just give out like that?

That was the last time I dislocated my left knee. Six months (or in this case an "eternity") had passed between the first injury and the fourth dislocation. The majority of it I spent in pain—or tensed up in anticipation of pain—all while losing a bit of faith in my body's ability to get me around like it used to. Believe it or not, I did not seek help for the dislocations and pain until after the fourth injury. I was frightened of what I might hear and dreaded learning the truth about what was causing the pain. After four dislocations, though, I finally pulled my head out of the sand and scheduled an appointment with a physician.

■ ■ ■

"The Truth is a Bitter Pill to Swallow."
~ Unknown

Chapter 4

MY WORST NIGHTMARE

A week later, Dr. Ellis, an orthopedic surgeon for the University of Louisville's sports teams, confirmed that I had completely torn my ACL, the Anterior Cruciate Ligament, in my left knee. That was the first time I got my knee checked out. Up to that point, I was afraid to know the truth about what was going on with my knee—I was afraid to find out if I needed surgery. After testing, Dr. Ellis confirmed my worst fear—the ACL in my left knee was torn and surgery was forthcoming. The surgery involved Dr. Ellis performing a patella replacement; the procedure included taking part of the patella (kneecap) tendon to replace the torn ligament; the ligament was attached with screws in the tibia (bone in my lower leg) and femur (bone in my upper leg). The goal of this surgery is to recreate the torn ligament so my knee wouldn't dislocate anymore.

Physical therapy is standard medical protocol after orthopedic surgery. Dr. Ellis prescribed several months of physical therapy and said once my left leg was within 80% of the strength of my right leg, I could begin working back to "normal" activities. In my mind, once I had the surgery and physical rehabilitation, I figured I'd be able to get back to competing in my first love, Judo.

Shortly after surgery and during physical therapy, I was fitted for a Don Joy® knee brace. If you aren't familiar with this brace, it is a big blue titanium knee brace that is designed to support and hold the knee joint in place. Basically, as part of standard protocol, I was fitted with this brace to make sure I didn't "undo" the surgery. Though the brace was supposed to offer some sort of support and protection, I felt very stiff and awkward in my body. The knee still hurt like hell and presented bizarre symptoms: for instance, the surgical scar would sweat. The rest of my body was fine, but the scar would sweat? I liken the way I felt post-surgery to an adolescent teenager—I felt goofy, uncomfortable, and had no idea what my body was doing. Even with the knee brace, I didn't feel much like exercising from a physical perspective. Mentally, I wanted to bike and run like I used to so I could get back into "Judo" shape. Every time I would start to exercise, the knee would begin to bother me or I would pull a muscle in my back. Something in my body would be screaming loudly telling me to stop. It felt like I was stuck between a rock and a hard place. I badly wanted to exercise and get the building tension and aggression released, yet there was no physical outlet for me without getting myself into more pain.

Three months later, the physical therapy was over, and I was deemed "good to go" by my doctor. However I still had pain, swelling, tension, and discomfort in my left knee, as well as in the rest of my body. There were still awkward compensation patterns going on in my feet, ankles, hips, and lower back as my body tried to "protect" my knee. I had to acknowledge the reality: I was still in pain and a dishearteningly long way from being healed and practicing Judo.

■ ■ ■

ACTION STEP:

Subscribe to my YouTube channel,
http://www.YouTube.com/TheKneePainGuru,
where you will find important information in videos
I have created over the last five years.

Chapter 5

THE JOURNEY TOWARD PAIN RELIEF

I found out through lots of research that even though I was in my early thirties, I was on a long path that would end in another surgery to replace my knee joint. Yes, really! Even though I'd endured two years of pain since my first knee dislocation, I had avoided pain medications and cortisone shots. But going the conventional medical route of physical therapy, drugs, and injections almost guaranteed an accelerated pace to knee-replacement surgery. That was (and still is) the standard protocol used when there is chronic pain with no resolution: replacing the knee joint.

Knowing that I had proceeded as far as I could with the medical model, I began to pursue "alternative" therapies to get some physical relief for how my knee and body felt. Some of the more common alternative approaches were massage therapy, Rolfing®, acupuncture, acupressure, Reiki, hands-on healing, healing touch, and chiropractic. All of these therapies offered relief for a period of time, but the effects would not last and the pain would return. There seemed to be something going on with my body, on a deeper level, which no single modality of healing (Eastern or Western medicine included) was able to remedy.

I couldn't believe the information that I was coming across in my research and in talking to clients. It didn't make sense to me. We have been born with the most amazing healing machine of all time: our body. Why are doctors going in and replacing parts of it with plastic and metal? I intuitively knew that this autopilot journey to surgery just couldn't be right. There had to be another way out of the downward spiral of pain, tension, and discomfort in the knees that lead to knee-replacement surgery. With all the options available to us, there MUST be something we are not looking at, are overlooking, or have not considered.

"Although I'm a knee surgeon, I have always believed that surgery should be your *last* option, not your first," says Dr. William Stillwell, Instructor of Orthopaedic Surgery at the College of Physicians and Surgeons of Columbia University. "If you suffer from chronic knee pain, first try a conservative, natural, holistic and non-operative approach. You have nothing to lose, but the pain."

Chapter 6

MEDICAL MODELING

What I've found out during the past fifteen years since my initial knee injury (while getting myself out of knee pain and helping thousands of clients do the same) is that the "endgame" for the repeating cycle of chronic knee pain management is a slippery slope that leads to a knee replacement surgery. No matter what your diagnosis is—arthritis, bone on bone, patella knee pain, etc.)—the traditional medical model will end with total knee replacement. While you are waiting for this knee replacement, pain management is the current accepted treatment for chronic pain. But even if you prescribe to the pain management methods, you are not guaranteed to be out of pain after knee-replacement surgery. So there is no current medical model for eliminating pain, only managing it.

The current medical model looks at chronic knee pain through a very narrow lens, and your options are pretty limited and bleak if what they are offering doesn't work. If you show up with knee pain and "nothing" is wrong with your knee or you still have knee pain after surgery, you will be looking at the following options: prescription drugs, painkilling injections, physical therapy, or exploratory surgery.

The hope with prescription drugs is that the pain cycle between your brain and your knee will be interrupted enough that your pain will be gone after the drugs leave your system. This usually works best for acute pain, but it is not a sustainable strategy for long-term chronic knee pain.

Using prescription drugs to eliminate chronic knee pain is pretty much the same approach as getting cortisone shots in your knee. Numb the pain, put a "band aid" on it, and maybe the pain will go away by the time you've finished the prescription. The real problem with this scenario is your nervous system "ups the ante" each time by not feeling what is happening in your knee. If the strategy is solely to numb the pain, the nervous system is still prompted to scream louder with more pain. This equates to the pain getting more severe each time it comes back, requiring stronger and stronger painkillers. Repeatedly upping the med dosage is not working as a long-term strategy; it's creating more pain.

Without a doubt, pain medications, as a long-term strategy for chronic pain are not a good idea. This would be the equivalent of unplugging your car's check-oil light when it alerts you that something is wrong. Your car will run fine for a while, but eventually something more drastic is going to happen with your engine. Similarly, numbing your nervous system and increasing your tolerance for pain is the same as turning off the warning light on your body. Eventually, the meds will not work well enough to numb your pain, and your body will scream louder. A drastic measure, surgery, becomes likely—you've burned out the engine.

Painkilling injections function much like a prescription drug; they are just more localized to the area where they inject the drugs. I've worked with clients who have informed me that after three cycles, each several months apart, they have to stop because cortisone is a steroid.

When I work with clients, one of the most common things I hear is, "I'm going for a cortisone shot to see if it will get rid of my knee pain." The idea behind a cortisone shot is that it will numb the pain and the knee can heal while you're walking on it because you are not able to feel the pain. On a nervous-system level, this is breaking up the pain loop from the knee to the brain. When the cortisone wears off, you're hoping that the knee pain won't be there. If you're looking for a "band aid" to your knee pain issue and you can handle needles, then a cortisone shot might not seem so bad.

In my experience, physical therapy modalities are pretty standard exercises that are intended to get you out of knee pain with the theory that strong muscles will somehow create a healing environment for the other functioning parts of the knee. Specified sets and reps of leg raises, leg extensions, leg curls, and calf raises are done mindlessly to get you out of knee pain. There's no consideration for how the knee feels each step of the way—the mentality is to push through the pain. *Knees for Life* focuses on training you to be aware of the types of tensions and pains you're experiencing and understanding what to do with each particular type of pain in its own special way. Performing random repetitions and sets of physical therapy exercises can all too often create more pain. During my time in physical therapy, the goal was to make sure my left leg had the correct flexibility and strength within 80% of my right leg. This was the goal to be measured. The concept of being comfortable in the process was not even a reality.

It is my experience that exploratory surgery is completely unnecessary on the journey to eliminating chronic knee pain.

I have yet to hear anyone who has seen any benefit from exploratory surgery. The idea behind the surgery is that the doctor should be able to see if there's anything wrong with the knee in an X-ray, CT scan, or MRI. The exploratory surgery creates undue stress and tension in the knee, creating more pain in the end. From my perspective, if what is going on in the knee is so small that it can't be detected, then it's not a large enough mechanical dysfunction to warrant surgery to correct it. So why chance the risks of exploratory surgery for the chance that your knee pain might go away?

The reason why the doctor wants to do the exploratory surgery is to see if they can find something that's causing the pain, when, in reality, what's causing the pain are tiny little nerves the width of an eyelash being irritated from stress and tension in the joint. Exploratory surgery is not going to see stress and tension in the joint. It carries risks, and there is no guarantee that the doctor will find what is causing the pain. The odds are when the doctor is done scoping your knee, your knee pain is going to be worse.

Even alternative pain-relief treatment plans can be invasive and ineffective. A couple of years ago, I was living in Charleston, South Carolina, and found myself at a health fair. There were all sorts of booths at the fair sharing different approaches to health and healing in the body. One booth particularly attracted my attention; it focused around pain management. I asked the nurse behind the table what their approach was to addressing pain. She was very sincere when she told me that the doctor, who had been practicing medicine for more than 20 years, begins the treatment by first tracing the nerve to the source at the connection with the spine, and then they do a cortisone injection to stop the signal of pain from the brain to the part of the body that's feeling the pain.

I said, "Interesting ... but what happens when the cortisone either doesn't work—or wears off—and the patient still has pain?" The nurse said they would do that procedure up to three times, and if that doesn't work, the doctor would perform surgery to burn and sever the nerve so the patient doesn't feel the pain anymore. Now, on the surface, this seems like a wonderful thing that the patient wouldn't feel pain anymore, but what about the long term? We were born with those nerves for a reason: the nerves signal us when something is wrong. If we cut those nerves with the goal of eliminating the pain, yes, maybe the pain will go away in the short term. But what are we doing to our nervous systems in the long term that will show up and manifest in other ways? Is this sustainable, and will it improve our quality of life? I don't believe this to be the case.

What's important to understand about this approach to chronic knee-pain management is the current model is not designed to eliminate your knee pain. Its purpose is to manage your knee pain until you are old enough for knee-replacement surgery.

According to the Agency for Healthcare Research and Quality on The American Academy of Orthopaedic Surgeon's website, over 600,000 knee replacement surgeries are done in the U.S. every year. This trend rises year after year. The reason they are waiting until you are "old enough" is because the average life of a replacement knee joint that is plastic and metal is about ten to twenty years.

For more information on this topic, see:

www.orthoinfo.aaos.org/topic.cfm?topic=a00389

More often than not, the current medical model will keep you in this holding pattern of "pain management" long enough that they will only have to replace your knee one time before your "expiration date" (death).

I know this may sound crazy, but it's true. No matter what your age—whether you're in your twenties or seventies—the current model will have you in a holding pattern consisting of physical therapy, drugs, injections, and surgery until you are "old enough" to have a total knee replacement.

Unfortunately, the reality of the current model is very different from what your knees need. Otherwise, there wouldn't be so many people suffering from knee pain, waiting to get old enough to have knee replacement surgeries. The problem arises with the concept that strengthening the muscles in the legs will make your knee pain go away. There is some truth to this statement, however, from my perspective, very little. The idea is that there is an imbalance in muscle tension and by strengthening the "weak" muscles, you bring balance to the leg and the knee pain will go away. Think about this, though: it wasn't like you went to sleep and when you woke up in the morning, suddenly certain muscles in your legs had weakened and caused imbalance.

It makes more sense from a nervous-system perspective that something got too tight, thus creating the imbalance. So now if you go ahead and strengthen the "weak" muscles, you are now reinforcing a dysfunctional tension pattern in your legs, creating conditions where your knee pain gets worse. Numbers don't lie, and with so many people suffering with chronic knee pain, a new approach needs to be looked at for a solution to be truly found. In my estimation, conventional physical therapy is just not effective.

The current approach is the holding pattern—to wait and see. There is no understanding or monitoring of how the pain is moving and changing in the knee, taking the client experience into account. By the time you're in your fifties or sixties and hobble into the doctor's office, after you've been suffering for years or decades with severe knee pain, you'd believe anything they would tell you just to make the pain go away—even if it sounded as ridiculous as, "How about we cut the bones in your leg off and replace it with plastic and metal?" It sounds crazy now, but believe me, it makes complete sense when you find yourself in that situation. You can make very strange choices under severe stress and pain.

I recently started working with Ben from Boulder, Colorado—he has had four knee surgeries. The last three were exploratory to look for something "wrong," and the pain in his knee has worsened each time. He finally got fed up with the "holding pattern" and decided to work with me because I have a solid strategy for him to get out of pain in the next three months, focusing specifically on creating a new reality of comfort in his knee.

The strategy is pretty simple and straightforward. We create as much comfort in the knee as possible with specific stretches that work with the subtle intrinsic movements in the knee joint. At the same time, we are setting up the conditions in Ben's life to make sure there is nothing in the way for his body to heal what is going on in his knee.

Do I believe that most doctors are well meaning in their attempts at helping you get out of knee pain? Yes. However,

I also believe the medical model only works when based on something in your knee being broken or torn. If you don't fit into that category, your best bet is to look at a more comprehensive, holistic approach to eliminating the pain you feel in your knees every day.

I prefer a more sustainable approach that seeks long-term relief. I like getting to the root cause of what is going on and having a deeper understanding of my body. That way, if the same issue presents itself again down the road, I will know what to do. Besides, I hate needles!

■ ■ ■

"When the only tool you have is a hammer,
you tend to see every problem as a nail."
~ Abraham Maslow

Chapter 7

A REAL PAIN IN THE KNEE

Whether you are reading *Knees for Life* before a medical visit or you've already had your visit and are puzzled by the diagnosis (or lack of a diagnosis), it is prime time to educate yourself on some important physical attributes of pain, how your body's nervous system reacts to pain, and how the current conventional medical model will likely steer you. You will learn that there is a radical difference in the medical model's goal of "pain management," versus the *Knees for Life* goal: *to eliminate your knee pain completely and permanently.*

Let's begin this discussion by asking you to consider your personal knee pain situation and which of the following two categories of knee pain you are in as you read this book:

1) You have knee pain, and something in your knee is broken or torn (mechanically wrong).

2) You have knee pain, and after a medical exam, you've been told "nothing is wrong."

If you find yourself in the first scenario, then your doctor will have a plan of action to address what is broken or torn (mechanically wrong) with your knee, such as a surgery to correct the mechanical dysfunction. After the doctor has corrected the problem with surgery, you will possibly find yourself in a new category where purportedly "nothing is wrong anymore." However, you may still find that your knee could be in a good amount of pain, causing you all sorts of symptoms, and you are just not enjoying your life like you want to.

Important: in either of these scenarios, it is important to visit your doctor and make sure nothing is mechanically wrong. There is a place for medicine, and there are times when surgery may be required.

In order to understand how your body will naturally heal, it's important to understand some physical properties of pain, how your body's nervous system reacts to pain, and what options are available for you to seek relief. The body experiences pain in two different ways: acutely or chronically.

-**Acute pain** is severe pain—the pain may follow surgery, trauma, or other conditions and diseases. Acute pain occurring in the first 24 to 48 hours after surgery is often difficult to relieve, even with medication.

-**Chronic pain** is pain that continues or recurs over a prolonged period, caused by various diseases or abnormal conditions. Chronic pain may be less intense than acute pain. The person with chronic pain usually does not display increased pulse and rapid respiration because these autonomic reactions to pain cannot be sustained for extended periods.

Regardless of whether acute or chronic pain is present, there are tiny nerve endings being irritated and sending a signal to the brain that you have knee pain. In order to eliminate this signal being sent to your brain, telling you that your knee hurts, the standard medical approach is to prescribe drugs or pain-killing injections to block the signal. If pain is really intense, we want to use pain meds sparingly. Initially, we want to have short-term strategies to help pain, with the longer-term strategy of eliminating pain. So in the first 48 hours, something to get you out of pain can be a good thing. After 48 hours, though, pain meds are only masking the issue. With my method, you can address the current pain and alleviate it naturally, moving forward to a place of comfort and optimizing the body's ability to heal.

Acute and chronic pain affect the nervous system in very similar ways. When you experience acute knee pain (less than 48 hours), you can take immediate action by using RICE therapy (Rest, Ice, Compression, and Elevation). I also would suggest you take some additional measures, like increasing water intake, altering your diet to eliminate gut-inflammatory foods like grains, dairy, and heavily processed foods, taking a magnesium supplement like Natural Calm®, and a supportive homeopathic both topically and sublingually, such as Traumeel®. However, once you are out of that first 24 to 48 hours and you've gotten your knee checked out by a doctor who's determined that "nothing is wrong," then you are looking at chronic pain, and we need to continue setting up the conditions so your body is able to heal itself quickly and efficiently.

Chronic pain (longer than 72 hours) really makes it challenging to allow your body to begin to heal itself. Think of it like a siren going off all the time when you are trying to sleep. Now imagine that siren going off inside of your body. When you don't sleep, your body naturally builds up with stress and tension. That stress and tension begins to put more pressure on the nerves in your body, including your knee, making your knee pain worse.

Unfortunately, being in a state of chronic pain stresses our nervous system around the clock—whether we are awake or asleep. Quite frequently, a source of insomnia is chronic pain, which only compounds the problem. The primary way your body is able to heal itself is through rest and recovery. If you don't address chronic pain stuck in the body, then you are setting up the perfect conditions for your body NOT to be able to heal itself.

Chapter 8

THE (VERY) NERVOUS SYSTEM

If you've been in the holding pattern of pain management, you've either been told by a physical therapist (or just started to believe yourself) that you need to push through the pain. The "no pain/no gain" or "push through the pain" mentality, coupled with your nervous system's response to chronic knee pain, sets up the perfect storm of conditions so your knees stay in pain for a long time. The body's natural response is to tense up.

In this state, your body physically starts to react to the pain responses by responding as follows:

- Squeezes out the synovial fluid in your joints

- Draws the water out of your bones

- Leaches minerals out of your system so your body can't absorb the water that you do drink

- Confuses the signals for thirst and food

- Slows down your metabolism/digestion

- Creates more of an acidic state in your body and increasingly irritates the nerves in your knee

The process of the body going into this type of fight-or-flight state sets up all the conditions required for you to have knee pain for the rest of your life, with the end result being knee-replacement surgery.

The Slippery Slope

Acute Knee Pain (24-48 hrs) --> Chronic Knee Pain (48 hrs <) - (Insert Your doctor's Diagnosis here) (Weeks, Months, or Years) --> Leads to degenerative changes, dehydrated joint, and arthritis --> Eventually bone on bone --> Knee Replacement Surgery

When your body is in pain, it goes into the Sympathetic State, which is the "fight or flight" mode, where the following happens:

Fight or Flight

- Heart rate increases

- Blood pressure increases

- Overall body tension increases

- Irritability increases

- Cortisol production increases (aiding in fat retention and diabetes)

- Body processes are slowed (metabolism, digestion, urination, defecation, possible weight gain)

- Body temperature control decreases (palms sweat)

- Electrolytes are lost at an unhealthy rate (including minerals such as sodium and calcium) which leads to a chronic state of dehydration, increased bone loss, increased chance of bone spurs and kidney stones

- Decreased sexual response/low libido/erectile dysfunction

- Pupils dilate (because you're always looking for the threat)

Rest and Relax

When your body begins to feel comfortable and relaxes, it goes into a Parasympathetic State, where it is able to rest and the following happens:

- Heart rate decreases

- Blood pressure decreases

- Overall body tension decreases

- Decreased irritability (in a better mood with family, friends, and loved ones)

- Decreased cortisol production

- Body processes increase/balance out (metabolism, digestion, urination, defecation, possible weight loss)

- Ability to control/normalize body temperature

- Retain electrolytes (sodium, potassium, and calcium)—ability to absorb water, retain/build bone mass

- Increased sexual response/blood flow to pelvis/increased libido for both men and women

- Pupils function normally (better eyesight)

In order to understand how the body holds tension, let's look at the concept called tensegrity structure, which was made popular by R. Buckminster Fuller.

Tensegrity structure: *The property of skeleton structures that employ continuous tension members and discontinuous compression members in such a way that each member operates with the maximum efficiency and economy.*

A simple way to picture tensegrity structures is that of a bicycle wheel. If you tighten/loosen up one spoke, it affects the tension in the rest of the bicycle wheel. Think of the last time you stubbed a toe. Your whole body compensated for your stubbed toe. In the same way, the tension in a bicycle wheel is affected by one spoke.

We can see many structures in the world that are tensegrity structures, such as the Epcot Center, bicycle wheels, and geodesic domes. The idea is that the tension in the structure is supported by the entire structure and is supposed to be distributed evenly throughout the entire structure. If excess tension is created in part of the structure, that tension affects the entire structure as a whole. In the context of knee pain, this means that the knees are the "weakest link" in the series of tension from the head to the feet. If we continue to strengthen the structure as it exists, like in conventional physical therapy, it further burdens the tensegrity structure and makes the tension and pressure on the nerves in the knee worse. This is why you will see such a fast progression of arthritis in someone's knees the more they have stress in their life, whether it be physical, mental, or emotional.

The really interesting thing about tensegrity structure (and your nervous system) is that when you create comfort in part of your body, it affects the entire tensegrity structure — so you are relaxing the entire tensegrity structure. This means we can have a very profound effect in very quickly relaxing not only the pain in your knees, but also in the rest of your body. It doesn't take a lot of time, energy, or effort to do so, just a little patience, the right mindset, and a willingness to look for the cues that your nervous system is switching over from a fight-or-flight response to a rest-and-relax response.

It's like learning to ride a bicycle; once you master it, you never forget how it feels.

Chapter 9

REALITY AND MISCONCEPTIONS

Based on my own personal experience, as well as my experience in working with thousands of knee-pain clients, I've discovered that there are three very significant misconceptions every person seeking relief carries:

Misconception 1: *It takes a long time to heal knee pain.*

Reality: If your approach is masking the pain with drugs and shots in the hope that your knee pain will go away and strengthening the muscles in the legs in the hope that knee pain will go away, then yes, you are correct, it will take a long time for your knee to heal, if at all. However, if you look at your body's response to knee pain on a nervous system level and get the pressure off the tiny little nerves the width of a human eyelash, while simultaneously setting the conditions (water, nutrition, stretching, breathing, and mindset) for your body to heal your knee pain, then your body will absolutely surprise you at the speed in which it is able to heal your knees.

Misconception 2: *It has to hurt to heal.*

Reality: Yes, knee pain hurts, and yes, it will hurt more if you are starting out with exercises to strengthen the muscles in the legs. By doing leg raises, leg curls, and leg extensions, you will most likely irritate the already inflamed and tender nerves in your knee. Whether or not your knees will heal at that point is highly questionable. However, if you choose to get rid of your knee pain by first getting the pressure off of the tiny little nerves in your knees, then the very next thing you are going to feel is comfort and relief because you are immediately eliminating the source of the irritation on the nerves causing your knee pain. So comfort is the key!

Misconception 3: *You have to work hard to get out of knee pain.*

Reality: Yes, if you believe that exercises are the first step in eliminating chronic knee pain, then you will have to work very hard. However, it is questionable whether or not you will ever get out of knee pain. But if you focus on creating comfort in your knee first, getting the pressure off of the nerves in your knee causing pain, while simultaneously setting up the other conditions (water, nutrition, stretching, breathing, and mindset) in your life to heal your knees, then getting out of knee pain will be easier than you ever thought possible. To be honest, the hardest part to getting out of knee pain is reframing the mindset that you have to work hard to get out of pain. Most people will even disregard the results they get from my program because it is so easy. In a way, the mentality is they almost don't deserve to "get away" that easily.

Chapter 10

THE THREE TENANTS

With my own injury, rather than consider another surgical procedure (knee replacement), I elected to focus on changing my mindset and believing that comfort could be achieved within myself. I had researched, found relief from pain, and found success working with others by combining three principles simultaneously. Each of these principles relies on specific behaviors, activities, and actions, depending on the level of pain being felt at a precise moment in time.

Knees for Life operates under the framework of three basic, yet intertwined, principles:

1) *Shift your mindset*

   Just like a businessperson or a professional sports player, your mindset and attitude toward extreme success will play a pivotal part in your success.

2) *Understand and give attention to your nervous system*

   Your nervous system acts and reacts to pain within your body and creates tension. Tension is directly opposed to relaxation, and in order to heal, the body must be in a state of rest and relaxation and be nourished to optimize your nervous system's responses.

3) *Operate from a place of comfort in your body*

> Initially, it will seem like a very foreign concept to experience comfort because we live in a society that pushes a no pain/no gain philosophy. When you are experiencing pain, your nervous system goes into a fight or flight mode. In order for healing to progress, we have to set up the conditions so the nervous system can switch into a rest/relaxation mode. Your reality will have to switch from one of experiencing pain to one of experiencing (and expecting) comfort. There will be no "pushing through the pain." I will equip you with the ability to experience a new reality: comfort.

Sounds easy enough, right? Believe me, it will not be easy at first. Some of the changes will be easy for you, some will seem far too simple, and some may require you to make some changes that you resist. Where most programs to eliminate knee pain begin, my program ends. Why? Because the first thing we have to do to get you out of knee pain is to get you out of knee pain.

Chapter 11

MINDSET

I believe the most important obstacle to overcoming chronic knee pain is your mindset. Numerous motivational experts (for example, Dale Carnegie's *How to Stop Worrying and Start Living* and *How to Win Friends and Influence People*, and Napoleon Hill's *Think and Grow Rich*) dedicate their careers to coaching toward a positive mental outlook and demonstrate how critical this outlook is in order to achieve goals. Many rich, famous, and powerful people use a positive mental outlook to achieve wealth, fame, and power. We can use the very same tools to move ourselves closer to eliminating chronic knee pain from our lives.

It is important to understand how the body works and how it can work against us when trying to achieve that goal. Our amydygla, or what I refer to as the "lizard brain," is the oldest part of our nervous system and part of our brain. It reflexively controls our nervous system's response to threats. It responds immediately to knee pain and can leave us functioning like a two year old when the pain gets too much. That's why you don't feel like yourself: your stress level rises as you constantly feel the pain in your knee.

(Reference Daniel Goleman: Emotional Intelligence)

How does the "lizard brain" work in relationship to healing chronic knee pain? And how important is a positive mindset as your knee begins to get better?

Take a look at the following example of my work with Bob.

My client, Bob, a 62-year-old tennis player, was limping when he first came to see me because of his elevated pain level. We were only into our second week when I received the following feedback from him:

Bill P (me): How are the activities I gave you from last week working for you?

Bob: Fair ... I can't bend my knees enough to comfortably get to the bottoms of my feet ... I could never do "the yoga sit" lotus. My knees stick way up in the air.

Me: Okay, so you shared what isn't working ... now tell me how the work I gave you last week has changed what is going on in your knee?

Bob: It is getting stronger ... changing shape (less swelling), despite a fair amount of activity—I moved a wood pile, worked in garden—mind you, slowly ... consciously. Whenever it feels weird, I sit back at the computer and do the twist to the left thing and the pull into the hip thing ... I am also starting to sleep better and for longer periods of time.

Me: Perfect! We will get that loosened up more this week ... I just need to know that it's changing ... you'll be playing tennis full out before you know it!

■ ■ ■

This type of response is quite common when knees begin to get better. Our amygdyla—or lizard brain—is designed to protectively react and keep us safe from danger. When we are experiencing knee pain, we perceive danger as being anything that causes pain in the knee. So the more we move, the more we perceive the danger everywhere around us. While it *is* self-protective, our lizard brain also will keep us from changing; we are "hardwired" in some ways *not* to get out of pain. As you can see from Bob's feedback to me, he is *remembering* (getting hung up in past feelings/experiences) what still hurts and what he cannot do.

As part of our healing process, we have to develop the mindset of "the glass being half full" and recognize what we are able to do right now, as we move forward to living our lives free of knee pain.

■ ■ ■

"We can't solve problems by using the same kind of thinking we used when we created them."
~ Albert Einstein

Chapter 12

OPERATING FROM COMFORT

The great news? Whatever your pain level is right at this moment, you can move from that point, into less and less pain, to a point of comfort – immediately.

I view knee pain very simply. Tiny eyelash-sized nerves in the knee being squeezed, signaling to your brain that you have knee pain. Short, sweet, and simple. Anything more complicated than this simple explanation detracts from our goal of getting you out of pain. I see so many people, including doctors, complicating the process with diagnoses of X-rays, CT scans, and MRIs. A diagnosis is nothing more than a doctor's educated guess at what they see on a "picture." The images are valuable to the extent of determining if something is broken or torn, but absolutely useless in getting someone out of knee pain quickly. Getting the pressure off of the nerves in your knee is the priority: no pressure = no pain.

Let me take you through this process—really drive home the fact that wherever you are in pain, you can move from that point into less and less pain, to a point of comfort – immediately.

Here's Steph's experience with knee pain and moving through this process:

Bill sharing the hands-on methods drove home the point that comfort can be felt immediately and pain can start to leave the body immediately. I'd had pain and swelling in my right knee for over six months. It prevented me from doing all my favorite activities. It was horrible, especially since it caused me to be dropped from my volleyball team.

I had an MRI scan, and the doctor told me that I would need exploratory surgery and that the main diagnosis was a crack in the kneecap and some sort of cyst. By then, this knee pain has stopped me from doing all sports, dance, and any other physical activity, and was leading me toward surgery (as the doctor recommended). But I wasn't interested in conventional methods that lead to prescription drugs, surgery, injections, and worse.

I sought out help from Bill, and he explained his process to me. He said it's vital to be totally present and listening to the body while using his methods, which requires each person to recognize where they are with their own knee pain at that very moment in time! That was pretty profound. He assisted me with a series of passive stretches, asking me where the pain was and how and when it hurts. I explained it hurt when force was applied forward-inward and forward-outward (both with passive and active pressure). He asked me to be present while he applied pressure in different directions – and to let him know how it felt at that moment in each direction.

At first, my response was "so you want me to tell you when it hurts normally – like when I get out of the car or when my leg gets caught on something?" and he said that this is exactly what you don't want to think about. He said to think about now – what is happening in how I am feeling right now. I then brought my attention to the pressure he was applying at that moment and was able to clearly describe how my knee felt, where pressure was, what kind and strength of pain was present, and where pain and pressure was not. He explained how comfort in a normally pain-filled knee is found. Then after a series of passive stretches, he re-checked the pressure in the directions that were hurting and asked me how they felt, and I was able to respond that they were not hurting in those directions or that there was some trace of the current pain still felt, then we would re-adjust the passive stretching, and then re-check for pain again, and it was gone. Very exciting, to say the least. I had just experienced the application of passive stretching – which takes the body only to a position of comfort, a key aspect of Bill's program.

What is your greatest misconception regarding your knee pain? It's probably either that you'll live forever with the pain or the only solution to your pain is an eventual surgery. That's a BIG misconception. And it's simply NOT correct!

I believe the body has an infinite capacity to heal itself. It knows how to pump blood and oxygen throughout your body without your involvement, it knows how to digest food, it knows how to eliminate waste, it knows how to relax and rest. So when the healing is not happening, we have to ask, "What is getting in the way of my body's ability to heal itself?" There are many factors to look at; some are very obvious, like stretching, exercise, and functional movement. Some are not so obvious, like water, food, proper breathing, and a positive mindset. However, they all play crucial roles, and we must collaboratively take all of them into consideration when trying to get out of chronic knee pain.

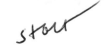

Chapter 13

SETTING YOUR GOALS

You are reading this book because you've decided you're not going to settle for a life filled with intervening pain management, you are not going to live in pain, and/or you want to avoid knee surgery. It's time to declare that you and your body will become pain free.

Yes, you are going to become pain free! Now, it is time to establish your goals.

One of the challenges in working with clients and picking a goal is they will have a huge laundry list of all the different things they would like to do and accomplish. Hiking, biking, walking, dancing, playing with their children or grandchildren, tennis, golf, etc.

So let's look at how to create a goal that is worth achieving. It needs to be specific and measurable. For example, I started working my client, Elena, in December, and she wanted to be able to run a 15K race in the middle of March and play a full match of tennis without thinking about her knees. This was a specific and measurable goal, and she was excited to get to work. We were able to tailor the work we did to achieve that goal, and we wanted it to happen in three months.

We didn't meet our goal. It did not happen in three months. It actually took her only seven weeks, and she didn't play three sets of tennis, she played four! Most people sell themselves short—they think they need to just tolerate and manage their knee pain and scale down their goals. In reality, if we completely alter our goals and adopt a new approach, knee (and body) pain elimination can be our new reality.

The key in choosing a goal is to pick the "first domino" that will tip over all the rest. This typically means picking the one thing you'd most like to do when you are out of pain. When I look back on the initial intake form from Elena, she made a list which included: "running, be more limber, strengthen quads, go up and down stairs, run a couple of marathons, exercise at the gym, play tennis, play in a tournament, wear high heels, avoid a knee-replacement surgery." This was quite a list.

As we talked through the list, I paid attention to what "lit her up," what she got excited about. This is key because what you are excited about is what is going to sustain and motivate you when the going gets tough. And it's guaranteed to get tough! But not like you think. It's tough mentally, and at the same time, you need to be gentle with your body while it progresses through its healing process. As your body heals and recovers more quickly, we can begin to push it more physically. However, you will know when this happens because there will be a sense of confidence and readiness that you can feel in your mind, body, and emotions.

Chapter 14

SETTING YOURSELF UP ⸌
TO SUCCEED

Before really digging into how we are able to completely eliminate the pain in your knees, we must first address one of the biggest obstacles. You've already done some challenging thought/mind work and dismissed the myth that knee-replacement surgery is the only option to get out of knee pain. The next (and biggest) obstacle is trickier — and once it is conquered, all other questions about addressing chronic knee pain will fall aside, as well. Setting yourself up to succeed is a mindset issue.

> *A fellow friend and Judo buddy, Dan, would tell me stories of how he got into fights when he was younger. Dan was small when growing up and didn't have any qualms about picking fights with opponents bigger than himself, not to mention with groups of people. He shared with me a strategy that I believe will be very useful. When faced with a group of people who wanted to kick Dan's butt, he would present the group with an offer for the toughest guy to step forward and he would fight him. More than once, everyone in the group would look at each other and decide that they weren't going to be the one to step forward and fight Dan – so no one fought.*

The idea is to tackle the toughest obstacle first; that needs to become your mindset.

For example, when the brain is thinking in a positive way, you will be able to focus on moving through the modalities, creating a state of comfort (and getting much-needed rest because of the improved, less tense, and more stress-free mindset!)

It's very important to focus on what is clearly positive and give little to zero energy to the negative.

How to state your intentions in your mind or aloud:

- I have comfortable legs
- I have strong knee joints
- I feel light and loose and free in my body
- I'm running a 15k easily
- I'm playing two sets of tennis by next month

How NOT to state your intentions in your mind or aloud:

- I have no pain in my knees
- I no longer have weak knee joints
- I don't feel stiff in my body
- I will run a 15k without pain
- I will play an entire match tennis without pain

See the difference? Words have power, especially the ones you say to yourself—don't use words like those listed above, that include "no, don't, without." Focus instead on using positive and healing words, like the proper statement of intentions: "I have, I am." This is so important!

■ ■ ■

EXTRA CREDIT:
Watch the movies "The Secret" and
"What the Bleep...Do We Know"

■ ■ ■

"The secret of change is not to focus on fighting the old,
but on building the new."
~ Socrates

■ ■ ■

"The jump is so frightening between where I am and where I want
to be ... because of all I may become, I will close my eyes and leap!"
~ Mary Anne Radmacher

Chapter 15

THE TOOLBOX

There are eight "tools" in your toolbox of relief and, just like tensegrity structures, if one of these tools is being underutilized, or not utilized at all, the likelihood of pain relief becomes less likely.

Modality #1: Mindset

There are certain tools that will span the three-principle spectrum in my practice, and some will be more mindfully or physically specific. You will find that your state of mind—your mindset—will be critical for all of them.

Tools for mindset advancement:

I'm a big proponent of a couple of tools to support a positive mindset when getting out of knee pain. One is the use of a Bach Flower essence called Rescue Remedy®. Many times, as the knee begins to bother us, we get bothered mentally, as well about the knee. Rescue Remedy® supports our body's ability to handle stress. There are times that just the stress in our daily life can cause the knee pain. Regardless of which it is, Rescue Remedy® supports our nervous system to let go of the stress and tension building up that is contributing to what is happening in our mind and contributing to our knee pain.

The next is journaling. In reality, I call it "Authentic Journaling." Back in 2000, I began my first journal. I wrote down what happened during my day, maybe listed the names of the people I met, the places I visited, and the things I saw. The journal in essence was pretty "sterile." I found I was censoring myself, thinking that I wouldn't want to have anyone read my journal in years to come and think poorly of me. As my life evolved, I realized how much this censoring affected the tension in my body. So I began using journaling as a means to vent the crazy thoughts that entered into my head. As humans, we are pretty irrational creatures that create all sorts of unnecessary tension for ourselves. "Authentic" journaling is a way to get this irrational stuff in our heads out and on paper—it gives the excess emotional and mental stress a place to banish ... it is no longer inside of us creating tension and contributing to our knee pain.

Here's what some "authentic journaling" looks like:

> *"How the hell did this happen? Why did I attract that experience into my life? What do I need to do to change that experience? It feels horrible, there's so much to do in my business and my personal life is all screwed up! I feel like screaming, like doing something. I used to go workout when I felt this way, until I screwed up my knee, then that aggression didn't work. Now what the hell do I do? My life feels like it's spiraling. Like it's not my own. How do I deal and function in integrity? There's such a rage I feel that seems misdirected and not serving me. I don't know what to do with it."*

As you can see, it's not pretty stuff, yet it bounces around in all of our heads and causes problems. If you are concerned about someone else reading the crazy stuff that comes out of your head, then you can burn the paper after you're done.

No muss, no fuss—everything is gone and out of you forever! You'll be surprised how much better you feel after you're done writing. You can either set a timer for 20 minutes and write as much as you can or just write until you're done, when it feels like there's nothing else to write down and bitch about. I find myself pretty exhausted after doing it. Try it and let me know how it goes and how you feel.

Modality #2: Hydration *Stuf*

I mention hydration foremost because it affects all three principles of *Knees for Life*: mindset, nervous system, and comfort. Hydration is key to keeping your mind and body functioning properly. To reach an adequate water intake level, you need to consume, in ounces, one-half of your body weight in water, per day (for example, a 200-pound person should consume 100 ounces of water). Just simple tap water. Simple, and it's important to be consistent and committed to doing this every day.

> **Tip #1**: Set a sixteen-ounce glass of water on your nightstand before you go to bed: the first thing you do the next morning is drink that water—you will already have started using one of the first tools in your toolbox and kick off your day already setting up the conditions your body needs to effectively heal your knees.

> **Tip #2**: Fill a pitcher with the number of ounces of water you need to drink every day. Mark the water level with a piece of tape. When the pitcher is empty at the end of the day, you know you've drunk enough water to make sure your knees can heal themselves.

Start fresh start

I remember working with a client, Janelle, several years ago, and she was not a big water drinker. We placed her on a program, and she was drinking her quota of water per day, and her knees were feeling pretty good. We were having a private consultation, and she told me how her knees were fine until she had her second cup of coffee. I said to her, "Good job noticing that; I like that you are noticing that difference." Even better, the next sentence out of her mouth was, "So I drank a couple of glasses of water, and my knee pain went away!" While drinking two glasses of water isn't going to be an automatic fix in every situation, it reminds us that hydration is a critical assistant in getting the nervous system to move from a state of tension to one of relaxation and being pain free.

There is a hierarchy for water allocation in your body. The brain and the blood dominate that hierarchy. If you are not hydrating properly, your body becomes dehydrated and draws water from your bones and the synovial fluid in your joints to make sure your brain and blood have adequate water to keep you alive.

This is one of the reasons why a dehydrated joint is one of the factors when a person is diagnosed with arthritis. (You will also find many people with similar conditions will also have bone spurs, osteoporosis, and calcified kidney stones.) A dehydrated knee joint is a beginning stage of arthritis. At this point of dehydration, even if you were to begin drinking plenty of water to hydrate your body and flush out your knee, you'll need the proper mineral content to supplement the hydrating properties of the water. I'd advise adding electrolytes (homemade "Gatorade") to your water consumption—these minerals will help the cells to absorb more of the water (and you won't be consuming more than your recommended ounces per day and running to the restroom too often!)

Recipe for the Original Gatorade:

One gallon of distilled water
Juice of one fresh-squeezed lemon
High-quality Celtic sea salt, one half to one tablespoon (to
taste)

I find the body's response to proper hydration pretty incredible. If you'd like to educate yourself further, I'd recommend reading *You're Not Sick, You're Thirsty*, as well as *Your Body's Many Cries for Water* by Dr. Fereydoon Batmanghelidj.

Modality #3: Nutrition

When I approach nutrition as a healing tool with clients, it is important that they have an understanding of the crucial priority to reduce inflammation. Many people have a mental image of inflammation – a cartoon-like throbbing gash or welt – which is a fairly accurate image when experiencing acute inflammation (a joint in the body gets twisted or otherwise injured, it swells, and is in pain.) Acute pain and acute inflammation are directly associated. What many clients have never learned is that the body can experience states of chronic inflammation that can severely inhibit our ability to remain in a state of progressive healing.

When it comes to healing and nutritional needs, your body has a hierarchy. When your body is trying to heal your knee, it needs the resources to do so. The knee joints are not that high in this hierarchy, what IS high are our "guts"... our intestines. When we eat foods that cause inflammation, primarily grains, dairy, and processed foods, it causes an inflammatory state in the intestines, and it can also cause discomfort, pain, and tension. At this stage of healing, the last thing you need is for your body to be "fighting off" irritating and inflaming foods. If your body is using close to 100% of its resources to heal the inflammation in your intestines, it has nothing left to heal what is going in your knee.

Pro-inflammatory foods like grains, soy, dairy, and processed foods need to be avoided and eliminated. For optimal healing, I have clients focus on organizing meals around nutrient-dense whole foods, like free-range and/or organic animal protein and organic vegetables. During the initial weeks of healing, I suggest minimal fruits (even sugar from fruit is inflammatory; cutting back is advised during healing process).

Talking about food can be a little tricky because there are so many thought processes, philosophies, and emotions associated with food, and they come with strong attachments—connected with family, nationality, religion, custom, comfort, and tradition. Most clients like working with as much information as possible, and the approach that I've found the most success with is typically referred to as "Paleo." If you don't like the word "Paleo," you can find another way to phrase it—nutrient-dense lifestyle, perhaps! Primarily, you'll be eating vegetables, lean animal protein, and healthy fats to keep the body properly fueled and minimize gut inflammation. I strongly recommend reading Robb Wolf's book, *The Paleo Solution*. Robb also has a very informative website. The word "Paleo" is bantered about a good bit lately, but in the healing realm, this nutrient-dense, whole-food-based lifestyle adjustment will result in less and less inflammation—and more and more healing.

If planning meals based on "real food" sounds either daunting or time consuming, consider a sample day's menu from my house. I keep it easy!

Breakfast:

> Four eggs
> Half avocado
> Half sweet potato

Lunch:

> Salad (Romaine, leaf, spinach)
> Olive oil/apple cider vinegar/fresh lemon
> Canned fish
> Nuts (cashews, almonds)
> Raisins
> Tomatoes
> Avocado

Dinner:

> Ground beef with onions and garlic
> Half sweet potato
> Half avocado or salad

■ ■ ■

"Let Thy Food Be Thy Medicine and Thy Medicine Be Thy Food."
– Hippocrates

■ ■ ■

Supplements

Questions concerning supplements are frequently asked, and, to be honest, we can (and should strive to) get the majority of our nutritional needs met if we are following the whole-food model previously described. Also, we should be mindful and make sure we are not eating foods that contain anti nutrients (compounds that leach nutrition out of our body faster than we can replenish). In times of severe pain/tension/stress, taking certain supplements can be beneficial. *Knees for Life* routinely updates our supplemental suggestions: visit www.KneesForLife.com/Supplements.

I personally use the following nutritional supplements to assist in times of stress, tension, or occasional pain.

Natural Calm® - Magnesium Supplement

Magnesium is typically one of the most deficient minerals in the human body. It is a laxative, so make sure you use it with caution—not enough will cause no change, and too much will have you running to the bathroom! Magnesium will help your body rest easier, and rest is crucial to a healing knee and body.

Rescue Remedy®

Helps with stress in the body and mental outlook. (See mindset section)

The combination of the following two Traumeel® products got me through fifteen years of abuse in Judo and my knee surgery.

Traumeel Gel®

Apply topically every ten to fifteen minutes when you have pain, until the pain begins to subside.

Traumeel Tablets®

Take sublingually according to the label to address pain, tension, swelling, and discomfort in your knee until pain begins to subside.

For the most comprehensive and updated list of Knee-Pain Guru nutritional supplements, please visit www.KneesForLife.com/Supplements.

Modality #4: Breathing

"Well if you don't breathe, you die..."
Systema Expert, Mikhail Ryabko when asked about
the importance of breathing.

■ ■ ■

Breathing is a tool to control our body's (and nervous system's) fight-or-flight response to pain, especially while moving in transition times, such as getting up from a chair, rising out of bed, and up from the floor. If we hold our breath, we tense up more, creating more stress in our body and setting up the conditions so our knees will hurt more.

We can hold our breath in minute ways, whether we are experiencing pain, tension, or emotional distress – regardless the body is tenser and more sensitive to feeling pain. A tense body will cause less space for nerves and lessens the body's ability to heal itself. Holding our breath creates more tension within our structure and ties directly into our nervous system. It's a very important part of operating from a place of comfort to breathe steadily through movements, to breathe steadily and mindfully if you are experiencing pain; the body needs the "help" of the breath to allow the parasympathetic/rest and relaxed state to move toward healing.

If your knee is hurting and you're afraid to move and holding your breath, you are actually making it more difficult for your body to heal itself due to the tension your body is holding. Even further, the breath deprivation causes tension/stress on your heart, lungs, and internal organs – the body is massaged by your breath; holding your breath stops that massage process. Not only is that holding up your healing process, but it's also where disease sets in.

Even if you're in pain, when you smooth out your breath, you begin to transcend the pain. As a result, you're reversing and relaxing the tension in your structure—now the pain isn't controlling pain; it's the breath that begins to control and relax the pain.

Let's look at a practical scenario that you can practice the next time you experience knee pain:

> *Assuming you are in a seated position, you rise to stand and begin to feel pain.*
>
> *Remember to slowly inhale through your nose, and exhale through your mouth with fully measured breaths. You may start increasing breaths as tension begins to increase, as smoothly and fluidly as you can, working with the breath to create the upward motion, until you are fully upright. This extra breath work might make you lightheaded, so make sure you're stable. You have done it: you've allowed your body to stay in a relaxed and healing place while standing and breathing through the discomfort. Good job! Now, remember how important hydration is and go drink a glass of water to further take care of your body's needs.*

Modality #5 Working in Comfort

"Make focusing on comfort your new reality."
~ Bill Parravano

■ ■ ■

We now reach the essence of my program, which is "make focusing on comfort your new reality." This section is the cornerstone of my approach, because here we are working directly with the stress and tension in the nervous system by creating comfort in your knee joint, by taking the pressure off of the tiny little nerves the width of a human eyelash that are sending a signal to your brain that you have knee pain. As we take the pressure off of the nerves in the knee, at the same time, we are paying attention to the cues in the nervous system that will tell us that a change is taking place in the knee.

■ ■ ■

ACTION STEP:
Get my FREE Report with four stretches to eliminate the pain in your knees:
http://thekneepainguru.com/free-information-report

Modality #6: Active Stretching

This section is putting the muscle under slight tension, being patient and waiting for the muscle to begin to let go of the tension on its own. Think of it like pulling taffy. If you pull the taffy too quickly, the taffy will snap and break. When applied to the muscles in your legs, that is not a good thing. But if you put the taffy under gentle tension, the taffy will begin to let go slowly and gradually stretch. What we are looking for is for the muscles in your legs to let go gradually to free up the tension your body is holding in your legs, hips, and back. All of that tension is being thrown into your knees, causing them to hurt.

■ ■ ■

ACTION STEP:
Get my stretching book, *The Comfort Zone*
www.thekneepainguru.com/lp/comfort-zone-stretches

Modality #7: Mobility—Neuromuscular Re-Education

When your body feels pain, it does a "work around." Like painting yourself into a corner, every time your body moves and feels pain, the range of motion your body is comfortable moving in gets smaller and smaller—you get into such a small place that you create more dysfunction for the joint. Your brain has to give your body the orders to work around pain, and the more you restrict and resist, you are teaching yourself a new way of dysfunctional movement.

Remember your "lizard brain" is designed to protect your body from getting injured further. By the time you are in a healing stage to incorporate mobility/neuromuscular re-education, you'll remember that all the previous modalities have strengthened and healed you this far. It is time to resist the urge to resist and restrict movements.

You can think of mobility work in the context of making your bed every morning. What has happened while you've slept at night is a series of twists and turns that have physically made a mess of the bed. In the morning, the bed needs to be straightened. Likewise, during the course of a day, you're typically going to go through the twists and turns of life. Most likely, you've restricted and used work-around movements and essentially ended up with a messy bed that needs to be made. When you do mobility work, you begin to straighten out all the twists and tangles and smooth out the stresses you've taken on during the day. The best part about mobility work is that it builds the confidence to know it is safe to move in certain ranges of motion, and your range of motion actually improves and increases as you continue the mobility work. Mobility work trains both your brain and your body to move and function more in balance and alignment with itself.

Modality #8: Exercise *Start*

Over 1,000 years ago, Marcus Tullius Cicero said, *"It is exercise alone that supports the spirits and keeps the mind in vigor."* I've liked this quote for quite some time, in part because Cicero's hometown, Arpino, Italy, was also the home of my great grandparents over 100 years ago. I also like it because almost every one of my knee-pain clients has had an ultimate goal to be mobile and active once they are pain free. Much has been learned about exercise since Cicero reminded us of the importance of exercise. In relation to the *Knees for Life* program, however, I believe the quote needs to be modified slightly:

Modified, the quote would read: *"It is **proper** exercise alone that supports the spirits and keeps the mind in vigor."* Before you started reading this book, if you were exercising and causing yourself more pain, you might have ended up in a pretty deeply depressed place. Fortunately, since we have worked the previous modalities to build a healthy body and operate going forward from a place of comfort, you should be feeling better overall by the time you are in the Stage Level Five, where we begin to exercise and become even stronger physically—and even more pain free.

If you've reached the exercise modality of the *Knees for Life* program, you are in a virtually pain-free place and will begin to build stronger joints, tendons, fascia, and muscle. Up until this modality, it has been important to ignore the social clichés of pushing through pain; instead, you've worked through seven other modalities to bring your body into a heightened state of health and relative strength.

As with the seven other modalities, it is important to keep your goals in mind. For me, the end goal is for you to have a strong, flexible, and healthy knee joint that lasts your lifetime. By nurturing our bodies and healing through the circumstances of comfort, we have set up the conditions so your knee joint is getting healthier by the day. Now we need to get it strong. Strengthening the muscles in the legs doesn't necessarily get the knee joint strong. We have to challenge the body in a certain way to make sure the joint gets the strength we are looking for.

Muscles fatigue after seven seconds. If you've ever watched a bodybuilder at the gym work his max bench press, as he starts to push up the bar, you could begin counting—one-thousand one, one-thousand two, one-thousand three—usually, if he does not get the weight all the way up in seven seconds, he's most likely not going to get the weight up. The muscles have fatigued by that time, so the only thing working are the tendons and ligaments in his arms and chest. The tendons connect muscle to bone, and ligaments connect bone to bone. After the muscles are sufficiently fatigued, you're working on strengthening your structure, and the body begins to shake when the muscles are sufficiently fatigued. What normally happens when the body is fatigued? We tend to hold our breath, quiver, and finally quit the exercise. That's working some muscle for you, but it is also ensuring that you have weak joints. The key for making sure you have strong knee joints is to fatigue the legs with body weight exercises, while making sure to breathe properly (revisit breathing section) and move slowly through the entire range of motion. This will guarantee you strong, healthy knee joints that last a lifetime, not to mention a strong body!

■ ■ ■

ACTION STEP:
Check out this video for an example of this type of exercise:
http://www.youtube.com/watch?v=bsAXfDvmPAQ

■ ■ ■

Once you are advanced far enough into the exercise modality, you will have developed the skills to nourish and hydrate yourself properly and should be operating from a place of comfort on a daily basis. Keeping momentum will require that you use a positive mindset to monitor your progress and mindfully tend to each of the previous seven modalities. Sometimes this will mean putting things off that will cause you pain. It's temporary!

SCENARIO 1

Let's say you decide to go for a run and your knee feels a little "twingey" when you start out. You think to yourself, *"I'll run through this, no pain no gain, right?"* So you do, you push yourself, and by mile 2, things are getting more and more painful. By the time you get home, your knee is painful and swollen. You take some Tylenol, do your RICE therapy, and think it will be better in a couple of days.

A week goes by, and your knee has gotten somewhat better but is still not back to normal. You decide to get it checked out by your doctor. You get an MRI, and everything turns up normal. The doctor gives you a prescription painkiller and sends you home. A couple of months later, you're running again, but your knee is still not quite the same. You see your doctor again, who suggests trying a cortisone shot or a series of three shots. You go through a series of those, and your insurance will cover you to go for physical therapy to strengthen the muscles in your legs.

That was a year and a half ago. Now, you're sitting in front of your doctor on the exam table, and he is suggesting an exploratory surgery to see if there's something the second MRI has missed. You decide to go for it. You get the report back from your doctor—he found some arthritis, cleaned that up, and discovered some narrowing of the joint. You tell the doctor, "Great, but I'm still in pain. What can I do?" He'll look at you and chalk everything up to old age. Ride your stationary bike and keep as active as possible.

This back and forth goes on for a few years with the doctor. You can't really seem to get an answer about why the pain keeps getting worse. You look into some of the new therapies and different injections to make the meniscus/cartilage regrow, you take your supplements MSM, glucosamine, chondroitin, but the situation only seems to be getting worse.

Now, the doctor is looking at you, saying your arthritis is getting worse and it's now bone on bone. You're a perfect candidate for a knee replacement surgery, but you're only in your fifties, so you have to wait until you are "old enough" to have a knee replacement surgery. Sound familiar?

SCENARIO 2

Here's how that same scenario could look like from a *Knees for Life* standpoint. You decide to go for a run, but your knee feels a little "twingey" when you start out. You think to yourself, *"How about I take a moment and feel the tension pattern my knee is protecting itself with and hold it in a position of comfort for a minute or two and see what happens?"* You do and as you're waiting for your nervous system to shift to a place of comfort, it comes into your awareness how stressed you've been lately, working extra hours and also arguing with your spouse more than usual.

You realize how much stress that has put your body under and if you decide to push yourself right now, things are only going to worse. You decide to walk a little bit, do a little mobility work, and head home for the day. You drink extra water and take it easy that evening. The next day, you wake up more rested than you've felt in quite a while and think, *"I'm ready for that run today!"*

Both scenarios start out the same, but the body awareness is very different. When you increase the awareness in your body, it's like setting up a better radar system that can pick up threats much further out, so those threats never get close enough to be a full-blown crisis. Paying attention to how your body feels is key.

Knee pain is created by a lack of awareness and understanding of what is going on in your body. Getting out of knee pain can only be truly done by creating more awareness and understanding of how to get yourself out of that pain.

■ ■ ■

ACTION STEP:
Get my exercise book, *Stop Your Knee Pain Now!*
www.thekneepainguru.com/lp/stop-your-knee-pain-now-4

Chapter 16

A ROAD GUIDE

Five Stages of Healing Your Knee Pain: Working the Program

To this point, we have discussed how critical your nervous system is to feeling and healing knee pain and how your body's tensegrity structure requires all operations to come together to function in a pain-free fashion. The understanding of the physical process is important to move into the healing modules: these modules will first ask you to evaluate your current pain level and then determine the order in which to use the tools from your "toolbox." Each day (heck, even each minute) has the potential to re-order your approach to pain.

You will have to learn (and practice often) to succeed. Let's sample different levels of pain you will be experiencing and the various steps to move through that particular level of pain.

What's Your Pain Level ... Right NOW?

When you're in pain, ask yourself, "What is my pain level at this moment?" There is no past or future when you are seriously going to eliminate chronic knee pain from your body. Every time we allow our mind to ruminate in the past pain, or worry about future pain, we "leave" the present and are not paying attention to what the body is telling us right now. Be honest with yourself—right now—and be present to what your body is feeling right now.

The danger of not listening to your body is that you will make your situation worse.

The benefit of listening to your body is the ability to have strong healthy joints that will last into old age.

So, ask yourself again, right now, "What is my pain level?" You're not letting your lizard brain sneak in, are you? We aren't talking about pain yesterday, tomorrow, five minutes ago, or five minutes from now—it's so easy for our lizard brain to get carried away in a whirlwind of lizard thoughts, like *"Sheesh, the pain was so awful last night before I went to sleep, so that means it's just going to get worse!"* The opposite can also be true—if you were doing really well and exercising two days ago and "now" your knee is really hurting, it's important for you to realize that you will begin that moment's module relative to the level of pain you are currently evaluating.

Looking at How You Feel

Your pain level is evaluated in *Knees for Life* similarly to how you were asked to assess your pain at a doctor's visit – a pain level of one being very little pain, a level five being moderate pain, and a pain level of ten being the most excruciating. Depending on where your pain level is currently, you will fall into one of the following five stages, and you can work through that stage's module.

Pain Scale of 1-10

Stage 1 – Pain Level 8, 9, 10 - Modules to focus on (Mindset, Water, Breathing, Food, Passive Stretching)

Stage 2 – Pain Level 6, 7, 8 - Modules to focus on (Mindset, Water, Breathing, Food, Passive Stretching)

Stage 3 – Pain Level 4, 5, 6 - Modules to focus on (Mindset, Water, Breathing, Food, Passive Stretching, Active Stretching)

Stage 4 – Pain Level 2, 3, 4, - Modules to focus on (Mindset, Water, Breathing, Food, Passive Stretching – as needed, Active Stretching – as needed, Mobility Work)

Stage 5 – Pain Level 1, 2 - Modules to focus on (Mindset, Water, Breathing, Food, Passive Stretching – as needed, Active Stretching – as needed, Mobility Work, Exercise)

So, let's work through a sample module. Have your lizard brain take a break (no worrying about yesterday's pain or the potential for any pain tomorrow). Determine your pain level right where you are sitting, *right now*.

Let's use the Stage-Two Module to illustrate the assessment and work that follows:

At Stage Two, your pain will be significant to severe. If you'll remember when we discussed the nervous system, it reacts to pain by tensing up to protect itself—it's important to be mindful of that and know that this is the time to ease yourself out of the tense sympathetic reaction your nervous system is setting up. A Stage-Two Module means focusing on your mindset (you will be out of pain soon), making sure you are breathing (deliberately in through the nose and out the mouth) and not holding your breath, assessing your recent intake of water and hydration level, considering your recent nutrition: are any of these things "off?" Remember: breathe.

Once conditions are met, you can move toward passive stretching for the specific type of pain you are feeling at that moment.

■ ■ ■

ACTION STEP:
✓ Get my FREE Report with four stretches to eliminate the pain in your knees:
http://thekneepainguru.com/free-information-report/

■ ■ ■

When pain drops to a four or five, you can move into Stage-Three and will add more passive and some active stretching exercises, such as quads, and hamstrings, and hips. When you are in pain, you are often sitting quite a bit because you are fearful of moving and feeling pain. The active stretching should feel really good and helps release some of the tension your body is holding.

When your pain drops more and you are in Stage Four, you will add neuromuscular reeducation and mobility work: you'll be moving your body in a controlled and systematic way that continues to help dissipate fear—you will become more confident in how your body is moving. The best part is you'll notice that you are feeling better in general. All the thoughtfulness and care you've given to yourself, the rest, the nutrition, and the proper hydration will have your body's healing well underway, and by not "pushing through the pain," you've ensured that you are healing properly.

When you reach Stage Five, you're not in much pain, and your body is ready to begin targeted exercises specifically to strengthen the tendons and ligaments in the knee itself. At this point, your knee will be ready to fatigue the muscles (to get them out of the way), then the body begins to work on tendon and ligament strength—it makes the joint, tendons, ligaments, and fascia very strong.

Re-evaluate Where You are Every Morning!

You will continue to measure your pain level in the morning and evening. You will consider that pain level each time, and that is where you move through that stage's module. It is a self-paced program, paced at the pain level your body is experiencing at the particular moment in time. It's what makes this program unique.

■ ■ ■

For more information about being present, check out *The Power of Now* , a book by Eckhart Tolle.

■ ■ ■

ACTION STEP:
Sign up for my program: Say No to Knee Replacement
www.SayNoToKneeReplacement.com

CONCLUSION

Bruce H. Lipton, PhD, was doing research on stem cells 45 years ago and his findings were so mind boggling that it changed his whole life and career path. Dr. Lipton is an internationally-recognized leader in bridging science and spirit, and he provides vital information about the power of the mind and healing. He's a stem-cell biologist, the bestselling author of *The Biology of Belief*, and recipient of the 2009 Goi Peace Award. Dr. Lipton has been a guest speaker on hundreds of TV and radio programs, as well as a keynote presenter for national and international conferences. The following is an excerpt from his welcome video on his homepage, where he shares some very important and heartfelt information about the power of the mind. (Hear it personally by visiting www.BruceLipton.com.)

"Did you know that we are essentially skin-covered petri dishes, and we have this built-in cultural medium called blood, and the composition of that cultural medium affects the state of the cells in our bodies (as demonstrated in my stem cell experiments)? It is most important to understand what controls the chemistry of your blood—which in turn controls your genetics and your behavior. The answer is in our perceptions of life!

The way we see life causes our nervous system to release chemistry into our brain: neuropeptides, hormones, growth factors, etc. This chemistry derived from the brain is actually added to the cultural medium of our body (blood), which in turn controls the fate of our cells! The very simple reality is: as you change your mind, as you change your belief, you change your biology! No longer shall we perceive ourselves as victims of heredity. Receiving genes that we didn't select, and genes that we can't change, and believing that these genes control our lives. We are totally empowered as masters of our biology. The way we see life, the way we respond to life, changes our genetics and our behavior, and also affects the way we live in this world! My sincere hope is for you to see how truly powerful you are in controlling your fate and the fate of the world in which we live."

Remembering always that we set the cultural medium for our own lives is how we will reach our goals. Our perspective, attitude, and persistence will carry us through to the end goal! Bruce Lipton couldn't have said it better — his research points to the data that portrays the same stem-cell makeup, in various cultural mediums, actually changes what is made based on the environment created. You created your own healing environment. Chemical changes can be affected by your intentions.

I want to repeat those last two lines, *"You created your own healing environment. Chemical changes can be affected by your intentions."* **We have both the intrinsic natural power and all the necessary tools to help our bodies heal. We just have to tap into that power and effectively utilize these tools.**

In closing, you may be sitting there overwhelmed, wondering, "What do I do next?" I just want you to know this is normal! This is your lizard brain, aka your nervous system, keeping you where you are—stuck with knee pain—just like millions of other people. Remember, the lizard brain is designed to keep us safe and out of pain AND protect us from change. In order for you to move out of pain to comfort, you are going to have to manually tell your lizard brain that everything is okay—it has done its job, but, for you to move forward at this point, it is no longer needed.

Now that you understand how your body works—on a more in-depth level—YOU take control of your destiny. This is exactly what this book is all about. Remember, there are three major points that you want to keep in the forefront of your mind!

1) Your mind is the biggest asset you have in eliminating your knee pain!

2) Comfort is the key to getting out of knee pain—the fastest!

3) A deeper understanding of your nervous system is absolutely what will guide you on your path to pain-free and healthy knees!

Now that you know the role that comfort plays in you getting out of knee pain, all you have to do is begin to focus on comfort—more than pain. We have talked about how it may seem difficult at first, but now that I have walked you through the concepts of how to apply comfort to your body, you know the pitfalls to look for as you begin. The more you practice this, the easier it gets! Comfort is your new best friend, your ally, your companion. Nothing else matters at this stage of the game.

Most important, you had to ignore what your body was saying to get you to the level of pain you are in now. This is a combination of how your nervous system is hardwired and how society has taught us to operate. The old "no pain, no gain" adage just doesn't cut it anymore! That's not even a long-term, sustainable, solution—it's merely a convenient response to a much more complex problem! The only way to get out of knee pain will be to shift your thinking and listen to your body, which will tell you exactly how to do it. It's not difficult in the sense that it takes a lot of effort; it's about shifting your thinking.

Now that you've completed the hardest part—understanding the concepts in this book and learning a new way to think—you're all set! All of this work is an accumulation of the past 14 years of my life and my dedication to helping people rid themselves of knee pain. The knowledge that you have now gained is the roadmap for your new journey to pain-free living.

Each of us is now a key player in this shift in thinking. Knee replacement surgery is no longer going to be the option for the majority of people. The exciting thing about this is once you're out of pain, you'll be able to share this with others, just like I have. I urge you to get involved and help others so they don't end up on the slippery slope of knee replacement surgery. Help empower each person to get a new lease on life. As my concepts work for you, they can be passed on and work for others, too.

My goal, as I have shared with you, is to eliminate knee replacement surgery in my lifetime. Please keep in touch, offer feedback, visit my website, share your victories and insights, ask questions, blog, and journal your success and lessons learned. I want to hear all about your journey. I'm here to encourage, support, guide, and continue learning right alongside you, and I'm honored to be on this mission together!

Please visit my blog for important discussions and feedback, my website for new information, my products page for the tools you will need along the way, my Facebook and Twitter pages so that we can network together, etc. As you know, the communication options are vast in this age of technology, so let's keep in touch. Send me feedback! I'd love to hear from you.

In closing, I want you to find that one thing in your life that you would be absolutely overjoyed to do if you didn't have to think about your knees: dancing, traveling, running, hiking, biking, or playing with your children or grandchildren. Let that be your motivation to make this happen. You can do this! Just be consistent and committed, and before you even realize it, your knees will be feeling better and you will be living the life you've always dreamed of. The very first sentence in this book reads: *My mission is to make knee-replacement surgery obsolete.* Every pain-free step you take is one step closer to making my vision a reality.

Here's to your strong and healthy knees—for life!

ABOUT THE AUTHOR

Bill Parravano is an international author, speaker, and teacher. Author of *Stop Your Knee Pain Now* and *The Comfort Zone*, he's been working with knee-pain sufferers since 1999. Bill has spent a tremendous amount of time researching pain management, pain elimination, and has a full working understanding of the body and all its movements. Bill uses a very "hands on" approach when it comes to working with his clients. His dedication is apparent in both his work and his attitude—he is extremely motivated to help others learn (and apply) their own body's healing potential. Bill has been applying an advanced understanding of Systema (a Russian Martial Art) in very relevant ways since the year 2000. The breathing techniques from this practice prove to be incredibly beneficial. Bill has completed over 2,000 hours of training in Ortho Bionomy®; this extensive training in body work has given him untold leverage when it comes to understanding the body and how it relates to pain. He has also studied the various movements of the body in order understand how movement affects change in the nervous system, which is an area of strong focus for Bill. His research has enabled him to help numerous clients reach their goal of becoming pain free.

Bill is not only a pioneer for alternative options to knee-replacement surgery, he is also breaking new ground when it comes to the natural healing of the body—and he has specialized in bringing this natural healing to the knees. Bill still spends much of his time in research and study, as the learning process never ends; he continues to apply cutting-edge techniques and methods as a result.

RESOURCES

EXPERT RESOURCES

Jesse Cannone:

Recognized as one of the leading back-pain relief experts in the United States, Jesse Cannone has been helping people eliminate their pain and regain control of their lives for more than a decade. He is an amazing example of how far passion, drive, and determination can take you. Jesse and I talk about how connected the body is and how the knees affect the back and the back affects the knees. In this interview, we discuss these important connections.

www.KneesForLife.com/Jesse-Cannone

Shawn Stevenson:

Shawn Stevenson is a Professional Nutritionist, specializing in biochemistry and kinesiological science, as well as advanced treatment for acute and chronic disorders. Shawn and I talk about the superfoods that can help re-grow the cartilage and meniscus in the knee joint. We cover several important super foods that aid in healing and rebuilding during this interview.

www.KneesForLife.com/Shawn-Stevenson

Dr. Frank King:

Dr. King is a nationally-recognized researcher, lecturer, and author in homeopathy. His passion to develop an innovative, highly efficient, and safe, natural medicine protocol launched him immediately into research following the establishment of his chiropractic practice. For over two decades, he and his colleagues have researched to discover the most successful natural medicines and their procedures. Dr. King has developed over 200 natural homeopathic medicines, along with new procedures, to empower both the physician and consumer in their quest for optimal health.

www.KneesForLife.com/Dr-King

Rob Brinded:

Rob has been working with elite sports for 15 years, with a variety of different sports from football to ballet. For the past six years, Rob has been working with Chelsea FC, where he had been working as a Rehabilitation, Strength and Conditioning Coach. After working with Chelsea, he set up his own company. Until 2009, he was contracted to work with a player from Barcelona FC. He is also an international health and conditioning consultant. Rob has a passion for movement and how movement can trigger reactions on a subconscious level. He is the author of *The Code of the Natural*. He discusses in detail the natural movement that can trigger attraction instantly and provides online exercise videos that release the body to move like it should.

www.KneesForLife.com/Rob-Brinded

Dr. William Stillwell ("Dr. Bill"):

Dr. Stillwell is a Fellow of the American College of Surgeons, the International College of Surgeons, the

American Academy of Orthopaedic Surgeons, and the American Academy of Neurological and Orthopaedic Surgeons. He is also a member of the Arthroscopy Association of North America, the Association for Hip and Knee Surgery, among numerous professional and scientific societies. In his professional work, he introduced a number of new surgical techniques and patient care innovations during his career, including the use of what eventually became known as clinical pathways and mega-dose intravenous vitamin therapy in the postoperative period after joint replacement. He lectured extensively to lay audiences and promoted community outreach programs to teach the public about medical issues. In the interview, Dr. Bill talks about the latest medical technology, how to regrow cartilage and meniscus, and other topics.
www.KneesForLife.com/Dr-Bill

Exclusive Resources for Knees for Life

Call the number on the front of the book; 877-891-9484, and listen to my recorded message.

Go to my website, www.KneesForLife.com, and sign up for my newsletter.

Follow me on Twitter:
www.Twitter.com/TheKneePainGuru

Connect with me on Facebook:
www.Facebook.com/TheKneePainGuru

Subscribe to my YouTube channel:
www.YouTube.com/TheKneePainGuru

Sign up for my program: Say No to Knee Replacement:
www.SayNoToKneeReplacement.com

Get my stretching book, *The Comfort Zone:*
www.KneesForLife.com/The-Comfort-Zone

Get my exercise book, *Stop Your Knee Pain Now!:*
www.KneesForLife.com/Stop-Your-Knee-Pain-Now

Suggested Reading List
www.KneesForLife.com/Book-Store

Mindset:

The Four Agreements - Don Miguel Ruiz
Loving What Is - Byron Katie
The Power of Intention - Dr. Wayne Dyer
What the Bleep Do We Know - Arntz, Chasse, Vincente
How to Stop Worrying and Start Living - Dale Carnegie
How to Win Friends and Influence People - Dale Carnegie
Think and Grow Rich - Napoleon Hill
The Power of Now - Eckhart Tolle
You Can Heal Your Life - Louise Hay
The 20-Minute Break - Ernest Rossi
The Power of Full Engagement - Tony Schwartz & Jim Loehr
Emotional Intelligence - Daniel Goleman
The Biology of Belief - Dr. Bruce Lipton
The Gift of Fear - Gavin De Becker
On Aggression - Conrad Lorenz
Lights Out: Sleep, Sugar, and Survival - T.S. Wiley with Bent Formby, Ph.D.
Uncertainty - Jonathan Fields

Water and Hydration:

The Hidden Message in Water - Masaru Emoto

You're Not Sick, You're Thirsty - Dr. Batmanghelidj
Your Body's Many Cries for Water - Dr. Batmanghelidj

Nutrition:
The Paleo Diet - Robb Wolf
Everyday Paleo - Sarah Fragoso

Breathing:
Let Every Breath - Vladimer Vasiliev

Passive and Stretching:
Relax into Stretch - Pavel Tsatsouline
Super Joints - Pavel Tsatsoulin